KRATOM MAENG DA FOR BEGINNERS

Unlocking The Power Of Kratom Maeng Da A Comprehensive Guide To Boosting Productivity, Alleviating Pain, And Achieving Balance And Emotional Well-Being.

Georgette Lockett

DISCLAIMER

The author of this book is not affiliated, associated, endorsed, sponsored, or approved by any company or individual. The views and opinions expressed in this book are solely those of the author and do not necessarily reflect the official policy or position of any entity.

The author hereby disclaims any relationship, collaboration, or partnership with any company or individual mentioned in this book. Any references to products, services, or individuals are provided for informational purposes only and should not be construed as an endorsement or recommendation.

Readers are advised to exercise their own judgment and discretion when applying the information provided in this book. The author shall not be held responsible for any actions taken by readers based on the content of this book.

This book is intended for general informational purposes only, and the author makes no representations or warranties of any kind, express or implied, about the completeness, accuracy, reliability, suitability, or availability of the information contained herein. Any reliance on the information in this book is at the reader's own risk.

The author reserves the right to update, change, or modify any information in this book without notice. It is the responsibility of the reader to verify any information before taking any actions based on the content of this book.

By reading this book, the reader acknowledges and agrees to the terms of this disclaimer.

Table of Contents

INTRODUCTION

Kratom, especially the Maeng Da strain, is widely used in traditional medicine and natural medicines. Maeng Da, which translates to "pimp grade" or "top-grade," is one of the most well-known and strong Kratom variations available in Southeast Asia, particularly Thailand. Its illustrious history is intertwined with cultural rituals and traditional medical treatments that span decades.

Understanding Kratom Maeng Da

Kratom, or Mitragyna speciosa in technical terms, is a tropical evergreen tree native to Thailand, Malaysia, Indonesia, and Papua New Guinea. For generations, indigenous people have chewed or brewed its leaves into teas for a variety of uses ranging from pain treatment to mood improvement.

Importance Of Kratom Maeng Da In Traditional Medicine

The Maeng Da strain has a major role in traditional Southeast Asian medicine due to its increased alkaloid content and peculiar characteristics. It is admired for its alleged potency and efficacy. Indigenous people have traditionally utilized it to relieve pain, increase energy, and improve mood, crediting it with characteristics useful for everyday living and particular therapeutic requirements.

Overview Of Kratom Varieties

Kratom comes in a variety of strains, each with its own set of properties, alkaloid profiles, and alleged effects. Maeng Da is distinguished by its high alkaloid content, including mitragynine and 7-hydroxy mitragynine, which is thought to contribute to its strength. Other strains, such as Bali, Borneo, and Malay, have variable concentrations of alkaloids, resulting in differences in their effects and potency.

The importance of Kratom Maeng Da in traditional medicine has sparked interest and usage well beyond its native areas, gaining worldwide attention. Its potential uses in current wellness practices, as well as continuous scientific research, have increased in popularity and demand.

Understanding the origins, cultural importance, and differences across Kratom types, including Maeng Da, gives a full understanding of its relevance, allowing for educated judgments and study of its possible benefits and hazards.

CHAPTER 1

History Of Kratom Maeng Da

Kratom Maeng Da, a highly strong strain of Mitragyna speciosa, has a rich historical and cultural heritage that is intertwined with its Southeast Asian roots.

Origins And Cultivation

Maeng Da, which translates as "pimp grade" or "pimp quality," originates in Thailand, one of the key cultivation areas for Kratom. Its distinct moniker denotes its excellent quality and potency. The exact origins of the breed are still a source of contention among aficionados. Some think it was created by selective breeding, while others believe it evolved organically. Regardless, it distinguishes itself from other Kratom strains by having a higher alkaloid profile and stronger effects.

Traditional Uses In Southeast Asia

Kratom leaves have long been used by indigenous civilizations in Thailand, Malaysia, and Indonesia for a variety of reasons. Traditionally, manual workers chewed these leaves to enhance energy and stamina during strenuous duties. Kratom was also utilized to relieve discomfort and control pain. Its consumption was strongly ingrained in the region's cultural traditions, ceremonies, and traditional medicine.

Evolution Of Kratom Maeng Da In Western Culture

Kratom became popular outside of its native areas in the late twentieth century. Maeng Da, in particular, piqued the interest of Western Kratom aficionados owing to its purportedly enhanced benefits. Its reputation for being more powerful than other strains drove increased demand and production.

The strain's distinct qualities, such as its alleged energizing and stimulating capabilities, drew consumers seeking a variety of advantages ranging from mood improvement to pain treatment.

Due to its categorization as a psychoactive chemical, Kratom faced several legal and regulatory hurdles as its popularity expanded in Western nations such as the United States and Europe. Despite this, Maeng Da remains a popular Kratom strain on the worldwide market, adored for its strength and distinct characteristics.

Understanding Kratom Maeng Da's historical path from its roots in Southeast Asia to its incorporation into Western societies helps contextualize its relevance and continued appeal among users seeking its stated benefits.

CHAPTER 2

Botanical Characteristics Of Kratom Maeng Da

Kratom Maeng Da, a distinct strain within the Mitragyna speciosa family, stands out for its powerful qualities, potency, and complex chemical profile. Understanding its botanical properties is essential for comprehending its cultivation and its consequences.

Botanical Classification

Kratom, technically known as Mitragyna speciosa, is a cousin of coffee plants and belongs to the Rubiaceae family. The Maeng Da variety is known for its distinct characteristics, which are said to be the consequence of selective breeding for increased alkaloid content and potency. The name of this strain translates to "pimp grade" or "best grade" in Thai, stressing its high quality.

Growth Conditions And Habitat

Kratom Maeng Da flourishes in Southeast Asia's tropical climes, particularly in Thailand, Malaysia, Indonesia, and Myanmar. It prefers rich, fertile soil, high humidity, and a warm climate. Its development needs ample sunshine, steady rainfall, and a soil composition that drains well. Kratom trees may grow to be up to 80 feet tall in their native environment, with thick, dark green foliage.

Leaf Morphology And Color Variations

Kratom Maeng Da leaves have different features. They're elliptical, shiny, and dark green. The prominence of prominent veins that vary in color, commonly red, green, or white, is one distinguishing feature. These vein colors often correlate to distinct alkaloid compositions, which may influence the effects of the strain.

• **Red vein Maeng Da:** Used for pain alleviation and relaxation.

• **Green vein Maeng Da:** Known for its balanced effects that provide both stimulation and relaxation.

• **White vein Maeng Da:** This kind is said to be more invigorating and energetic.

Variation in vein color and leaf pigmentation results in variances in alkaloid content, which may have a considerable impact on the strain's potency and possible effects on humans.

Understanding these botanical qualities aids in the cultivation and identification of genuine Kratom Maeng Da, as well as assuring optimum growing circumstances and supporting users in picking strains that fit with their desired effects.

CHAPTER 3

Chemical Composition

Kratom Maeng Da is well-known for its powerful effects and distinct chemical profile. Understanding its chemical makeup entails diving into its active chemicals, which are predominantly alkaloids, and contributing to its qualities and effects on the body.

Active Compounds In Kratom Maeng Da

Over 40 alkaloids have been found in Kratom leaves so far. The particular composition and concentration of alkaloids may vary depending on several circumstances, including the age of the plant, the environment, and the processing processes used. The alkaloids found in Maeng Da, such as mitragynine, 7-hydroxy mitragynine, paynantheine, and speciogynine, are said to be particularly strong and numerous.

Alkaloids And Their Effects

1. Mitragynine is the most prevalent alkaloid found in Kratom leaves. It functions as a partial opioid agonist in the brain, binding to opioid receptors. Mitragynine adds to the stimulating and analgesic benefits of Kratom intake.

2. 7-hydroxymitragynine: This alkaloid is regarded as one of Kratom's most powerful constituents. It has analgesic benefits and contributes to the calming effects noticed in certain Kratom strains, making them more soothing.

3. Paynantheine and Speciogynine: These alkaloids are found in lower concentrations than mitragynine and 7-hydroxy mitragynine. While their specific methods are unknown, they are thought to modify some of Kratom's effects and may contribute to its overall influence on the body.

Impact Of Environment On Alkaloid Levels

Various environmental conditions impact the alkaloid concentration of Kratom, including Maeng Da. Soil composition, temperature, altitude, and even the precise geographical region where the Kratom is grown may all have a substantial influence on alkaloid levels. Kratom growing in various places, for example, may have varied alkaloid profiles, resulting in diverse effects.

The plant's growth rate, alkaloid output, and overall potency may all be affected by environmental factors. Because of its renowned potency, Kratom aficionados often recommend that Maeng Da be farmed under certain circumstances or undergo selective breeding to increase certain alkaloid concentrations.

Understanding Kratom Maeng Da's chemical makeup is important for customers since it aids in anticipating its effects and directing dose recommendations. However, it's important to remember that scientific research on Kratom, particularly its unique alkaloid profiles and effects, is still underway, and more research is required to completely appreciate its complexities.

CHAPTER 4

Effects And Benefits

Physical Effects On The Body

Kratom Maeng Da, noted for its potency, may cause a variety of bodily consequences. Among these impacts are:

• **Pain Relief:** One of the main reasons for Kratom's appeal is its analgesic properties. Because of its interaction with opioid receptors, it may help reduce chronic pain disorders.

• **Energy Boost:** Maeng Da is well-known for its stimulating effects, which provide consumers with more energy and alertness. Some users claim increased physical stamina after ingestion.

• **Relaxation and Muscular Relaxant:** Unlike its stimulating qualities, Maeng Da may produce relaxation at lower dosages, possibly relieving muscular tension and encouraging relaxation.

Cognitive And Psychological Impact

Kratom Maeng Da's cognitive and psychological effects might vary depending on dose and individual response:

- **enhanced Focus and Mental Clarity:** Users often report enhanced mental clarity and focus after drinking Maeng Da, which may lead to higher productivity.

- **Mood Enhancement:** Due to its interaction with neurotransmitter systems, Kratom Maeng Da may have mood-enhancing effects. It may reduce anxiety symptoms and produce a feeling of well-being.

- **Euphoria and Sedation:** At larger dosages, Maeng Da may cause euphoria and sedation. Users should proceed with care since bigger dosages might amplify these effects.

Therapeutic Uses And Potential Benefits

Kratom Maeng Da has been linked to several putative medicinal advantages, including:

• **Pain Management:** Because of its analgesic effects, it is popular among those looking for alternate pain reduction solutions for chronic diseases.

• **Anxiety and tension Relief:** Due to Maeng Da's relaxing qualities, several consumers report lower anxiety and tension levels after eating it.

• **Mood Regulation:** Kratom Maeng Da may offer antidepressant-like effects, possibly assisting persons suffering from mood problems.

• **Opioid Withdrawal Aid:** According to anecdotal evidence, some people use Kratom, particularly Maeng Da, to alleviate opioid withdrawal symptoms. More study, however, is required to substantiate these assertions.

While these effects have been claimed by users, individual experiences might vary greatly, and scientific research supporting these claims is relatively scarce.

Before utilizing Kratom Maeng Da for therapeutic reasons, like with any drug, take caution and contact a healthcare practitioner.

CHAPTER 5

Consumption Methods

Kratom Maeng Da, a well-known strain recognized for its strong effects, may be ingested in a variety of ways. Consumption methods differ from traditional to contemporary, with each altering the onset, intensity, and duration of its effects. Understanding these routes of ingestion is critical for users to make educated dose and experience selections.

Traditional Preparation Techniques

1. Chewing the Leaves: Traditional users of Kratom in its native areas often chew fresh Kratom leaves. This form of direct ingestion allows for the slow release of alkaloids into the circulation. This strategy, however, may not be possible for individuals living outside of the native areas owing to a lack of fresh leaves.

2. Brewing Kratom Tea: Brewing Kratom Maeng Da leaves or powder to make tea is a popular traditional practice. This process extracts the alkaloids into the water, making them simpler to consume. It is popular because of its simplicity and ability to control flavor.

3. Chewing Kratom Leaves with Betel Nuts or Other Enhancers: In certain cultures, Kratom leaves are chewed with betel nuts or other substances to improve the experience or alleviate its bitterness.

Modern Consumption Practices

1. Toss and Wash technique: This technique includes mixing Kratom powder with a liquid, often water or juice. It's a simple yet fast process, however, some may find the flavor and texture problematic.

2. Many users choose Kratom Maeng Da pills or tablets for their ease. These provide accurate dose

levels and are a discreet method to ingest Kratom without having to cope with its unpleasant taste.

3. Mixing with Food or drinks: A common way to hide the flavor of Kratom powder is to mix it with food, smoothies, or drinks. It may be made more appealing to consume by combining it with yogurt, juice, or a protein smoothie.

Dosage Guidelines And Considerations

• **Begin with Low Doses:** It is recommended that beginners begin with a minimal dose, often between 1 and 2 grams, to test individual tolerance levels and sensitivity.

• **Gradually Adjusting dose:** Users may gradually raise their dose by modest increments based on individual reactions and desired outcomes. However, excessively large dosages must be avoided to reduce any side effects.

- **Tolerance and Sensitivity:** Over time, regular users may acquire tolerance, needing greater dosages to get the same results. To control tolerance, it is advised to take pauses or practice rotation.

- **Avoiding Excessive usage:** Excessive usage of Kratom Maeng Da might cause nausea, dizziness, or drowsiness. It is critical to select an ideal dose that balances the intended benefits without going too far.

Understanding these methods of consumption and dosage considerations is critical for safe and enjoyable Kratom Maeng Da use. Before selecting a preferred mode of intake, users must educate themselves on appropriate consuming habits and consider personal characteristics. Consultation with healthcare experts or experienced users might give useful insights and direction.

CHAPTER 6

Safety And Precautions

Potential Risks And Side Effects

1. **Digestive Issues:** Some Maeng Da kratom users may have digestive issues such as nausea, vomiting, or constipation, particularly when taking greater dosages.

2. **Dependency and Withdrawal:** Like other kratom strains, regular use of Maeng Da may lead to dependency and subsequent withdrawal symptoms after ceasing usage. Irritability, mood fluctuations, muscular pains, sleeplessness, and anxiety are all possible withdrawal effects.

3. Long-term and excessive usage of Maeng Da has the potential to develop into addiction. Individuals with a history of drug misuse may be more prone to developing a kratom addiction.

4. Psychological Effects: Higher dosages of Maeng Da may cause hallucinations, disorientation, or agitation in certain people.

Interaction With Other Substances

1. Interactions with other drugs or medicines: Kratom Maeng Da may interact with other substances or medications, especially those that influence the central nervous system. When Maeng Da is used with drugs such as alcohol, benzodiazepines, or opioids, the risk of unpleasant effects or respiratory depression increases.

2. Medication Interactions: Kratom may interfere with the metabolism of some pharmaceuticals in the liver. Before using Maeng Da, it is critical to contact a healthcare provider, particularly if you are using prescription drugs.

Safe Usage Practices And Recommendations

1. **Controlled Dosage:** Begin with a minimal dose of Maeng Da to assess its effects on your body. Increase the dose gradually as required, but avoid taking overly large quantities.

2. To reduce the possibility of reliance or tolerance, it is best not to ingest Maeng Da on a regular or routine basis. To avoid possible addiction, space out consumption.

3. **Quality and supplier:** Make certain that the Maeng Da you buy comes from a reliable and trustworthy supplier. Contaminated or contaminated kratom might have negative consequences.

4. **Monitoring Your Health:** Evaluate your health regularly while utilizing Maeng Da. If you experience any odd symptoms or adverse effects, stop using the product and seek medical attention.

5. Pregnancy and Lactation: Due to insufficient study on its effects in these settings, it is highly suggested that pregnant or lactating women avoid consuming kratom, particularly Maeng Da.

6. Minors and others who have a history of drug misuse should avoid taking Maeng Da kratom.

Before introducing Maeng Da or any other kratom strain into your regimen, always talk with a healthcare practitioner or qualified specialist, particularly if you have pre-existing health concerns or are using drugs. Understanding the possible hazards and using Kratom Maeng Da with caution might help you have a safer experience.

CHAPTER 7

Legal And Cultural Aspects

Legal Status In Different Countries

• The legal status of kratom differs greatly across nations. Some countries prohibit its sale, possession, or usage, while others permit it with varied degrees of control. In the United States, for example, the legal status of kratom differs by state. It is important to understand the individual rules and regulations in each location.

Cultural Significance And Traditions

• Kratom has long been utilized for medical and cultural uses in Southeast Asian nations such as Thailand, Malaysia, and Indonesia. For ages, it has been used in religious rituals, cultural customs, and as a traditional cure.

Current Regulatory Landscape

• The regulatory environment for kratom is changing. Several nations continue to dispute its legal position owing to differing perspectives on its possible advantages vs hazards. Before deciding on legal status, government health organizations often assess its safety and potential for misuse. There are continuing debates in certain places to develop criteria for its safe usage.

Understanding these characteristics is essential for understanding the legal and cultural environment that surrounds Kratom Maeng Da. When addressing Kratom, it's critical to highlight careful use, adherence to regulatory standards, and respect for cultural customs.

CHAPTER 8

Research And Studies

Kratom Maeng Da has certainly gained notice in scientific and academic circles. While much study is continuing, the present knowledge of its effects and prospective applications has been explored.

Scientific Research On Kratom Maeng Da

Composition of Alkaloid:

Several studies have been conducted to determine the precise alkaloid content of Maeng Da Kratom and how it varies from other strains. Because of their possible biological consequences, the quantities of mitragynine and 7-hydroxy mitragynine, among other alkaloids, have been a focus.

The pharmacological activities of Kratom Maeng Da have been studied to better understand how its alkaloids interact with opioid receptors and neurotransmitter systems in the brain. The unique mechanisms of action compared to typical opioids have piqued the curiosity of researchers.

Pain Control:

Kratom Maeng Da's analgesic qualities have been studied, notably its potential for addressing chronic pain problems. Some study shows that it may help with pain relief via modulating opioid receptors.

Withdrawal and Addiction:

Investigations on Kratom Maeng Da's addictive characteristics have been undertaken, offering insight into its potential for dependency and withdrawal symptoms.

Researchers are seeking to determine how addictive it is in comparison to standard opioids.

Clinical Trials And Findings

Efficacy Research:

Clinical studies have been conducted to assess the effectiveness of Kratom Maeng Da in a variety of situations, including pain treatment, mood improvement, and possible assistance in opiate detox. These studies are aimed at determining its efficacy and safety for human ingestion.

Assessments of safety:

Several studies have been conducted to analyze the safety profile of Kratom Maeng Da, including its possible side effects, ideal doses, and risk of dependency. These results are critical for developing safe use recommendations.

Future Prospects And Areas Of Study

Considerations for Regulation:

Ongoing study adds to the ever-changing regulatory framework that surrounds Kratom Maeng Da. The findings of this research will very certainly influence rules and legislation governing its legality and availability.

Applications in Medicine:

Beyond its traditional usage, further study into Kratom Maeng Da may reveal further medicinal potential. Understanding its methods of action may lead to the development of innovative treatment strategies.

Long-term Consequences:

Long-term research is required to evaluate the long-term usage of Kratom Maeng Da, shining light on any cumulative effects, health hazards, or advantages linked with long-term intake.

As research progresses, a thorough knowledge of Kratom Maeng Da's pharmacology, effectiveness, and safety is anticipated to emerge, providing insights into its potential in a variety of medicinal and therapeutic applications.

CHAPTER 9

User Experiences And Testimonials

Personal Accounts Of Kratom Maeng Da Usage

Kratom Maeng Da offers a wide spectrum of user experiences because of its powerful and unique characteristics. People from many walks of life have shared their own experiences, putting light on the varied ways in which Kratom Maeng Da has changed their lives.

1. Pain Control and Relief:

Many users have claimed favorable results while utilizing Kratom Maeng Da for pain relief. Individuals suffering from chronic pain disorders such as arthritis or back pain have found relief by using this specific Kratom strain. Maeng Da's alkaloids are thought to interact with the body's receptors, providing a natural alternative to standard pain treatment approaches.

2. Stress Reduction and Improved Mood:

Another recurring topic in customer feedback is the mood-enhancing benefits of Kratom Maeng Da. Following intake, users often report an improved mood, greater energy, and a general feeling of well-being. This has inspired some people to include Maeng Da in their everyday routines, particularly during times of stress or low vitality.

3. Enhancement of Cognitive and Focus:

Several users have emphasized Kratom Maeng Da's cognitive advantages. Commonly stated benefits include increased attention, mental clarity, and concentration. This has led to the usage of Maeng Da by those looking for a natural cognitive boost for work, school, or artistic endeavors.

4. Therapeutic Applications and Potential Benefits:

Kratom Maeng Da has been studied for its medicinal potential in addition to its recreational usage. Some users have claimed good results in treating anxiety and depression symptoms. However, it is important to remember that individual reactions may vary, and Kratom's effects on mental health are still being studied.

Varied Experiences And Perspectives

1. Variations in Dosage:

Users often underline the need to determine the best dose for their requirements. Some people claim that lesser dosages provide the best results, while others prefer a greater amount. Among the parameters determining the appropriate dose are personal tolerance, body weight, and individual biochemistry.

2. Timing and duration:

Another aspect that influences Kratom Maeng Da ingestion is the time of day. Some people like it in the morning for an energy boost, while others prefer it in the evening for relaxation. The length of effects may also vary, with some users claiming a longer duration than others.

3. Personal Sensitivities:

Users' sensitivities and responses to Kratom Maeng Da might vary greatly. While some people may enjoy excellent outcomes with little side effects, others may be more sensitive and should use care while adjusting their dose. Understanding one's unique sensitivities and beginning with smaller dosages is frequent advice.

Finally, the user experiences and testimonies of Kratom Maeng Da demonstrate the adaptability of this botanical drug. However, it is important to use Kratom carefully, taking into account individual variances and being educated about possible hazards and advantages.

CHAPTER 10

Sustainability And Ethical Considerations

Due to increased demand and commercialization, Kratom Maeng Da, like many other natural resources, confronts issues in terms of sustainability and ethical concerns. This chapter dives into many areas of environmental effect, ethical sourcing, and conservation and responsible use programs.

Environmental Impact Of Kratom Harvesting

- **Biodiversity worries:** As demand for Kratom grows, there are worries about its influence on biodiversity. Overharvesting in specific areas may disrupt local ecosystems, harming a variety of plant and animal species.

- **Deforestation:** Uncontrolled or irresponsible harvesting techniques may result in deforestation, threatening the natural habitats of Kratom plants. This has the potential to significantly upset the natural equilibrium of these areas.

Ethical Sourcing And Sustainable Practices

• **Responsible Harvesting Techniques:** It is critical to promote sustainable harvesting techniques. This entails putting laws in place to guarantee that Kratom is collected in a way that does not hurt the environment or local populations.

• **Fair Trade and Labor Practices:** Ethical issues also include fair remuneration and working conditions for people participating in the Kratom business, ensuring that workers are paid fairly and work in safe locations.

Initiatives For Conservation And Responsible Usage

- **Conservation Programs:** Collaborative initiatives including local communities, governmental authorities, and conservation groups may aid in the establishment of conservation programs. These programs seek to safeguard Kratom ecosystems and encourage environmentally friendly harvesting practices.

- **Educational Campaigns:** It is critical to raise knowledge about sustainable practices among Kratom consumers and stakeholders. Positive improvements may be brought about by educating customers about responsible consumption and the need to support ethical and sustainable sources.

Challenges And Prospects For The Future

• **Regulation and Compliance:** Balancing the demand for Kratom while maintaining sustainable practices necessitates appropriate regulation and compliance mechanisms at both the local and international levels.

• **Research and Innovation:** Investing in research and innovation allows for the exploration of more ecologically friendly growing techniques. Exploring strategies to increase Kratom's advantages while limiting its environmental effect is also a possible future growth path.

The long-term viability of Kratom Maeng Da is strongly reliant on responsible methods, conservation measures, and ethical sourcing. To maintain the sustainability of Kratom and the well-being of the ecosystems and populations it affects, it is critical to balance financial interests with environmental and ethical issues.

Conclusion

We've gone into the complex world of Kratom Maeng Da throughout this tutorial, learning about its history, composition, effects, and many uses. Let us review the important findings and ponder the relevance of this floral gem while looking forward.

Recap Of Key Points

Kratom Maeng Da, a powerful strain of Mitragyna speciosa, is notable for its high alkaloid content, particularly mitragynine, and 7-hydroxy mitragynine. These chemicals bind to opioid receptors and have a variety of effects on the body and mind, ranging from pain alleviation and mood improvement to possible medicinal uses. Its classic and contemporary applications provide a wide range of sensations and effects.

Summary Of Kratom Maeng Da's Importance

Kratom Maeng Da's importance stretches beyond cultural and traditional bounds. Its diverse benefits appeal to those seeking pain relief, mood enhancement, and possibly medical aid. Furthermore, it piques the interest of academics, paving the way for possible applications in the medical and wellness areas.

The history of Kratom Maeng Da, from its indigenous beginnings to present consumption behaviors, exhibits a unique blend of tradition and adaptability. Its worth is derived not just from its effects, but also from the cultural significance and experiences of its users, who have provided a range of testimonies that have shaped our sense of its potential.

Looking Ahead: Future Of Kratom Maeng Da

As we look forward, the legality, research, and sustainability of Kratom Maeng Da are at an interesting juncture. Continued scientific research is required to reveal its full potential, allowing for appropriate usage and knowledge of its consequences.

However, this future is complicated by ethical concerns. Preserving its habitat, using sustainable harvesting procedures, and embracing ethical sourcing will be critical in guaranteeing the sustainability of Kratom Maeng Da without jeopardizing ecological integrity or threatening indigenous populations who rely on it.

With its rich past and complicated pharmacology, Kratom Maeng Da draws us into a world of possibility and possibilities. Understanding the complexity, advantages, hazards, and ethical implications of this botanical miracle is critical for full enjoyment and responsible use.

As we come to the end of this guide, may it serve as a compass, leading people, researchers, and policymakers toward educated judgments, ethical practices, and a balanced approach to maximizing the potential of Kratom Maeng Da.

The adventure does not stop here; it is an invitation to continue exploring, practicing sustainable habits, and learning about this amazing floral marvel.

THE END